Postherpetic Neuralgia

A Beginner's Quick Start Guide to Managing Shingles Through Diet, With Sample Curated Recipes

mf

copyright © 2022 Patrick Marshwell

All rights reserved No part of this book may be reproduced, or stored in a retrieval system, or transmitted in any form or by any means, electronic, mechanical, photocopying, recording, or otherwise, without express written permission of the publisher.

Disclaimer

By reading this disclaimer, you are accepting the terms of the disclaimer in full. If you disagree with this disclaimer, please do not read the guide.

All of the content within this guide is provided for informational and educational purposes only, and should not be accepted as independent medical or other professional advice. The author is not a doctor, physician, nurse, mental health provider, or registered nutritionist/dietician. Therefore, using and reading this guide does not establish any form of a physician-patient relationship.

Always consult with a physician or another qualified health provider with any issues or questions you might have regarding any sort of medical condition. Do not ever disregard any qualified professional medical advice or delay seeking that advice because of anything you have read in this guide. The information in this guide is not intended to be any sort of medical advice and should not be used in lieu of any medical advice by a licensed and qualified medical professional.

The information in this guide has been compiled from a variety of known sources. However, the author cannot attest to or guarantee the accuracy of each source and thus should not be held liable for any errors or omissions.

You acknowledge that the publisher of this guide will not be held liable for any loss or damage of any kind incurred as a result of this guide or the reliance on any information provided within this guide. You acknowledge and agree that you assume all risk and responsibility for any action you undertake in response to the information in this guide.

Using this guide does not guarantee any particular result (e.g., weight loss or a cure). By reading this guide, you acknowledge that there are no guarantees to any specific outcome or results you can expect.

All product names, diet plans, or names used in this guide are for identification purposes only and are the property of their respective owners. The use of these names does not imply endorsement. All other trademarks cited herein are the property of their respective owners.

Where applicable, this guide is not intended to be a substitute for the original work of this diet plan and is, at most, a supplement to the original work for this diet plan and never a direct substitute. This guide is a personal expression of the facts of that diet plan.

Where applicable, persons shown in the cover images are stock photography models and the publisher has obtained the rights to use the images through license agreements with third-party stock image companies.

Table of Contents

Introduction 6
Varicella-zoster Virus and Postherpetic Neuralgia 8
What Are the Symptoms of Postherpetic Neuralgia? 10
How to Diagnose Postherpetic Neuralgia? 12
When to See a Doctor? 14
    Who is at risk of getting postherpetic neuralgia? 14
What Are the Medical Treatments for Postherpetic Neuralgia? 17
How to Prevent Postherpetic Neuralgia? 19
Managing Postherpetic Neuralgia Through Home Remedies 21
Managing Postherpetic Neuralgia Through Diet 27
    Foods to Eat 27
    Foods to Avoid 32
Sample Recipes 37
    Baked Flounder 38
    Asian-Themed Macrobiotic Bowl 39
    Chicken Salad 41
    Baked Salmon 42
    Asian Zucchini Salad 43
    Low FODMAP Burger 44
    Stir-Fried Cabbage and Apples 45
    Asparagus and Greens Salad with Tahini and Poppy Seed Dressing 46
    Roasted Chicken Thighs 47
    Arugula and Mushroom Salad 48
    Fresh Asparagus Salad 49
    Tuna Salad 51
Conclusion 52
References and Helpful Links 54

Introduction

Postherpetic neuralgia (PHN) is a disorder that can manifest itself in a patient after chickenpox. The chickenpox virus, which causes the itchy, blistering rash we associate with a childhood disease, remains latent in the nerve cells of a person after they have recovered from the disease. Shingles are the result of the virus becoming active again, which can happen in certain people.

When nerve cells are injured as a result of shingles, a condition known as postherpetic neuralgia can develop. The end outcome is persistent discomfort in the area that was afflicted. The discomfort can range from moderate to severe, and it may linger for several months or even several years.

There is currently no known cure for postherpetic neuralgia; however, there are therapies that may assist in alleviating the pain associated with the condition. These include medical treatment, surgical procedures, and lifestyle changes.

In this quick start guide, we'll discuss in detail the following subtopics:

- Varicella zoster virus and postherpetic neuralgia
- What are the symptoms of postherpetic neuralgia?
- How to diagnose postherpetic neuralgia?
- When to see a doctor?
- Who is at risk of getting postherpetic neuralgia?
- What are the medical treatments for postherpetic neuralgia?
- How to prevent postherpetic neuralgia?
- Managing postherpetic neuralgia through lifestyle changes
- Managing postherpetic neuralgia through diet

So read on to learn everything you need to know about postherpetic neuralgia!

Varicella-zoster Virus and Postherpetic Neuralgia

Postherpetic neuralgia is caused by damage to the nerve cells that results from a previous infection. When these cells are damaged, they are unable to send signals properly, which can lead to the development of persistent pain.

Shingle is a condition that causes a painful rash. The rash typically appears on one side of the body and can last for several weeks. In some cases, the pain associated with shingles can linger for months or even years after the rash has resolved. This condition is known as postherpetic neuralgia.

Shingles are caused by the varicella-zoster virus, which is the same virus that causes chickenpox. The virus lies dormant in your nerve cells after you've had chickenpox. In some people, the virus reactivates as shingles. When the rash from shingles clears, the pain associated with postherpetic neuralgia can begin.

The varicella-zoster virus is a member of the herpesvirus family, which includes the viruses that cause cold sores and genital herpes. The varicella-zoster virus is spread through direct contact with the fluid from chickenpox blisters or through the air after someone with chickenpox coughs or sneezes.

You can't get postherpetic neuralgia from someone with shingles, but you can get chickenpox if you haven't had it before. After you recover from chickenpox, the varicella-zoster virus remains inactive in your nerve cells. In some people, the virus reactivates as shingles.

What Are the Symptoms of Postherpetic Neuralgia?

PHN is diagnosed when people have pain for more than 30 days after the shingles rash has healed. The pain can be severe and debilitating, interfering with activities of daily living. PHN can last for months or even years. Some people experience recurrent episodes of PHN. Some of these symptoms include:

- Chronic pain: The pain associated with postherpetic neuralgia can range from mild to severe. It is often described as a burning, stabbing, or shooting pain. The pain can be constant or intermittent. It may be worse at night. The pain is usually limited to the area where the shingles rash occurred. In some cases, the pain can spread to other areas.
- Numbness: You may feel like your skin is numb or tingling.
- Sensitivity to touch: You may be sensitive to even the lightest touch, such as from clothing.

- Allodynia: This is when you feel pain from stimuli that don't normally cause pain, such as a gentle breeze.
- Hyperalgesia: This is when you feel an exaggerated pain response to stimuli that would normally cause pain.

Postherpetic neuralgia is a painful illness that can develop in people who have had shingles in the past. Pain that lasts for more than a month after the rash caused by shingles has cleared up is a hallmark symptom of postherpetic neuralgia (PHN). The pain can be described as searing, agonizing, stabbing, or throbbing, and it might be confined to one location of the body or extend across the entire body.

A person's quality of life can be substantially diminished by PHN, which can make it difficult for them to sleep, eat, and carry out other activities of daily living. There is currently no known cure for PHN; however, there are therapies that may be able to help alleviate the discomfort.

How to Diagnose Postherpetic Neuralgia?

The earlier postherpetic neuralgia is diagnosed, the more likely it is that treatment will be effective. Your doctor will take a thorough medical history and do a physical examination. In some cases, your doctor may order a blood test or skin biopsy.

Medical History: Your doctor will ask about your medical history, including whether you've ever had chickenpox or shingles. Your doctor will also ask about your pain, including when it started, how severe it is, and what makes it better or worse.

Physical Examination: Your doctor will examine your skin for a rash. They may also press on different areas of your skin to check for pain, tenderness, or numbness.

Imaging Tests: In some cases, your doctor may order imaging tests, such as an MRI or CT scan, to rule out other conditions that can cause similar symptoms.

Blood Tests: In some cases, your doctor may order blood tests to check for other conditions that can cause similar symptoms.

Skin Biopsy: In some cases, your doctor may order a skin biopsy to rule out other conditions that can cause similar symptoms.

After a thorough evaluation, your doctor will be able to diagnose postherpetic neuralgia and can start you on treatment.

When to See a Doctor?

It's always best to see your doctor if you're experiencing any sort of pain that lasts for more than a few days, interferes with your daily activities, or is accompanied by a rash. Once postherpetic neuralgia is diagnosed, your doctor will work with you to develop a treatment plan.

If you think you may have PHN, it's important to see your doctor as soon as possible. Early diagnosis and treatment can help to improve your long-term outlook.

Who is at risk of getting postherpetic neuralgia?

While it is not clear why some people develop PHN and others do not, certain things may increase your risk of getting this condition.

Age

One risk factor for developing postherpetic neuralgia is age. The condition is most common in people over the age of 60. This may be because the immune system weakens with age, making it harder for the body to fight off infections.

Additionally, nerve tissue deteriorates as we get older, which may contribute to the development of chronic pain conditions like postherpetic neuralgia.

While age is a risk factor for developing this condition, it is important to note that postherpetic neuralgia can occur at any age. Therefore, everyone needs to be aware of the symptoms and seek medical treatment if necessary.

History of shingles

A person's history of shingles is one of the largest risk factors for postherpetic neuralgia. To develop postherpetic neuralgia, a person must first have shingles. Therefore, having a history of shingles is the largest risk factor for postherpetic neuralgia.

Weak immune system

One of the most significant risk factors for postherpetic neuralgia is a weak immune system. When the body is unable to fight off infection, the likelihood of developing complications, such as nerve damage, increases. Individuals with HIV/AIDS, cancer, and other conditions that impair immunity are especially at risk.

In addition, people taking immunosuppressant medications or undergoing radiation therapy are also at increased risk for postherpetic neuralgia. In general, anything that weakens the immune system can make an individual more susceptible to developing this condition.

If you have a high risk for postherpetic neuralgia, it's important to see your doctor right away if you think you may have shingles. Early diagnosis and treatment can help to reduce your risk of developing this condition.

What Are the Medical Treatments for Postherpetic Neuralgia?

The goal of treatment is to relieve the pain and other symptoms associated with postherpetic neuralgia. While there is no cure for postherpetic neuralgia, there are several treatments that can help to ease the pain. Some of the medications for postherpetic neuralgia include:

Topical Cream: Applying topical cream or ointment to the affected area can help to soothe the nerve endings and reduce inflammation. Some of the topical medications that may be recommended include lidocaine, capsaicin, and baclofen.

Antidepressants: Tricyclic antidepressants, such as amitriptyline and nortriptyline, can help to relieve pain by interfering with the way pain signals are sent to the brain. These medications are usually taken at night because they can cause drowsiness.

Anticonvulsants: Medications, such as gabapentin and pregabalin, that are typically used to treat epilepsy can also be effective in treating postherpetic neuralgia. These medications work by reducing the number of pain signals sent to the brain.

Local Anesthetic: Applying a local anesthetic, such as lidocaine, directly to the affected area can help to numb the pain.

Steroid Injection: In some cases, a steroid injection may be recommended. This injection can help to reduce inflammation and pain.

Surgery: In severe cases, surgery may be recommended. This is typically a last resort option and is only considered when other treatments have failed.

However, it is important to note that postherpetic neuralgia can often be a chronic condition, meaning that symptoms may persist for months or even years. As such, it is important to work with a healthcare provider to find a treatment plan that works best for you.

How to Prevent Postherpetic Neuralgia?

Postherpetic neuralgia can be treated with medication, physical therapy, and other treatments. There are also some things that you can do to prevent PHONE from occurring.

Chickenpox vaccine: If you have chickenpox, it is important to get the vaccine. The chickenpox vaccine can help to prevent you from getting the virus in the first place. If you have already had chickenpox, the vaccine can help to prevent you from getting it again.

Consult a doctor immediately: If you have shingles, it is important to see a doctor as soon as possible. Early treatment can help to reduce your risk of developing PHN. One of the most important things to do is to prompt treatment for shingles as soon as possible. This can help to shorten the duration of the initial outbreak and reduce the chances of developing PHN.

Shingles vaccine: It is highly recommended that those over the age of 60 acquire the vaccination for shingles. You may reduce your risk of acquiring shingles by being vaccinated against the disease.

Avoid injuring your skin: If you are suffering from chickenpox or shingles, you should refrain from touching or scratching your skin. Additionally, you need to make sure that the afflicted region stays clean and dry. It is essential to refrain from causing any further damage to the skin around the rash. Use soap that is mild on the skin, and stay away from hot showers.

Wear loose-fitting clothes if you have shingles: If you have shingles, you should dress in comfortable clothing that does not constrict your movements so the rash can be cured correctly.

If you have shingles and are suffering nerve pain after an outbreak, you should talk to your doctor about strategies to manage your pain and limit the likelihood that you will develop postherpetic neuralgia.

Managing Postherpetic Neuralgia Through Home Remedies

Postherpetic neuralgia, sometimes known as PHN for short, is a condition that a person may get after suffering from shingles. Pain that continues for longer than three months after the rash caused by shingles has healed is the primary sign of postherpetic neuralgia (PHN). Even though there is no known treatment for PHN, there are certain home remedies that may assist in alleviating the discomfort and improve the quality of life for those who have the condition.

Chamomile oil

Chamomile oil, which possesses properties that make it anti-inflammatory as well as antibacterial, contributes to the healing process of ulcers and pressure sores by aiding in the production of new skin cells.

One of the most frequent treatments for wounds of this nature is to use chamomile oil topically. Chamomile oil is effective in reducing the symptoms of postherpetic neuralgia, a painful kind of nerve injury that can develop as a sequel to shingles. When administered topically, it helps to calm irritated nerves and promotes the healing process.

Eucalyptus oil

It has been shown that eucalyptus oil can successfully reduce inflammation. In addition, the oil extracted from eucalyptus can speed up the process of wound healing, particularly for open wounds. As a consequence of this, the essential oil of eucalyptus has the potential to be an efficient therapy for postherpetic neuralgia.

Tea tree oil

It has been established that tea tree oil, which is obtained by pressing the leaves of the *Melaleuca alternifolia* plant, has properties that are both anti-inflammatory and antibacterial.

Cold compress

It is possible that using cool compresses or cloths directly to the irritating areas of the rash would be beneficial. This will assist in minimizing the irritation, and there is a possibility that it will also give some relief from the discomfort. Additionally, to lessen the severity of the effects that PHN has on one's quality of life, it is essential to protect one's skin from being subjected to excessive temperatures.

Witch hazel

Because it possesses qualities that are both anti-inflammatory and analgesic, witch hazel can help decrease swelling and alleviate pain. In addition to this, the anti-itching properties of witch hazel can also alleviate inflammation.

As a consequence of this, it functions quite well as a therapy for postherpetic neuralgia. However, it is essential to keep in mind that witch hazel is not appropriate for everyone's skin type. It's possible that for some people, it makes their illness much worse.

If you are thinking about using witch hazel as a treatment for postherpetic neuralgia, you must see a medical professional first. They will be able to provide you with guidance on whether or not the therapy is appropriate for you.

Cool shower

The cooling effect of the water might assist in calming the skin and provide some relief from discomfort. Scrubbing the skin in the afflicted region, on the other hand, should be avoided at all costs because doing so might irritate the nerve endings, which will result in further discomfort.

It may be possible to maintain the region clean by lightly brushing the skin with a soft cloth. This should not cause any further discomfort to the patient. Those who are afflicted with this ailment may find that their quality of life is improved by taking chilly showers or baths daily, which can assist in lowering their chance of developing postherpetic neuralgia.

Oat Baths

Rehydrating the skin and calming irritation caused by dryness and sensitivity are two of the many benefits that come from using oat extract. In addition, the flavonoids and saponins that are included in oat extract may help in the process of reducing inflammation. As a consequence of this, taking a soothing bath with products that contain oats is likely to give some relief from the pain that is linked with PHN.

Gentiana scabra

Gentiana scabra is a flower that can be blue or purple and can be found all across North America. It has been demonstrated to have a good effect on the prevention of PHN and the relief of discomfort associated with shingles.

Diet

Carotenoids are a type of antioxidant that has been demonstrated to both strengthen the immune system and bring down inflammatory levels. Oranges, red peppers, tomatoes, spinach, and kale are examples of foods that contain a high concentration of carotenoids. If you have postherpetic neuralgia, including these items in your diet may help to alleviate the pain associated with it as well as enhance your general health.

Quit smoking

The immune system becomes more vulnerable to infection as a result of smoking, which is especially true in senior people. Smoking also reduces recovery and healing times. Consequently, if you are a smoker and suffer from postherpetic neuralgia, giving up smoking may be beneficial to your condition.

Manage stress

It is possible that engaging in soothing activities such as meditation and making an attempt to sleep should assist you in experiencing less stress. By assisting in the relaxation of both the mind and the body, meditation can be an effective method for providing pain relief. Attempting to sleep when you can also assist in lowering stress levels and improving your general mood.

Taking time off over the day to refresh and unwind is another helpful strategy for lowering levels of stress. By taking some time out of your day to relax, you can help lower your chance of getting postherpetic neuralgia.

You may help to enhance your quality of life and lower your risk of acquiring postherpetic neuralgia by adhering to these guidelines and reducing your risk of developing postherpetic neuralgia.

You must visit a medical professional if you are experiencing symptoms of postherpetic neuralgia. They will be able to provide you with guidance on the treatment that is most appropriate for your condition. It may be important to take medicine in some circumstances to successfully manage the pain. However, these home treatments can also help to alleviate the symptoms of postherpetic neuralgia.

Managing Postherpetic Neuralgia Through Diet

Diet is one of the most important factors in managing PHN. By making simple changes to your diet, you can help manage the pain of PHN and improve your quality of life.

Foods to Eat

Foods high in carotenoids

Carotenoids are a type of antioxidant that has been demonstrated to both strengthen the immune system and bring down inflammatory levels. Oranges, red peppers, tomatoes, spinach, and kale are examples of foods that contain a high concentration of carotenoids.

If you have postherpetic neuralgia, including these items in your diet may help to alleviate the pain associated with it as well as enhance your general health. Carotenoids are largely responsible for the coloration found in fruits and vegetables. They are located in the fatty tissues of the body and may be found in abundance.

Carotenoids, in addition to having antioxidant capabilities, also assist in protecting cells from harm caused by UV radiation, which is another benefit of these pigments. Even though the majority of individuals obtain enough carotenoids through their food, taking supplements can be an effective way to increase your intake. For instance, taking a carotenoid supplement may help to lower the chance of developing macular degeneration, a condition that can eventually result in blindness if left untreated.

Carotenoids are also being investigated for the possible function they might play in the prevention of cancer. However, before any firm conclusions can be reached about this topic, further study in this field is required. Nevertheless, increasing the number of carotenoids in your diet by eating foods that are rich in them is an excellent way to improve your health.

Anti-inflammatory foods

There is currently no known cure for postherpetic neuralgia; however, there are therapies that may assist in lessening the severity of pain and inflammation associated with the condition. Consumption of foods that are known to reduce inflammation is one kind of therapy. Salmon, olive oil, and broccoli are just a few examples of foods that have been shown to have chemicals that have been demonstrated to help decrease inflammation.

In addition, these meals provide a wealth of nutrients that are necessary for the maintenance of healthy nerves. As a consequence of this, consuming foods that are known to lower inflammation and pain may be beneficial in the treatment of postherpetic neuralgia.

Anti-inflammatory spices

Certain spices, in addition to the meals that are good for reducing inflammation, can also be helpful in this regard. One example of a spice that has been used for millennia in India due to its reputation for having therapeutic benefits is turmeric.

Recent research has found that turmeric includes chemicals that aid in decreasing inflammation. [*Curcuma longa* or turmeric] As a consequence of this, including turmeric in your diet has the potential to assist in the alleviation of the discomfort and inflammation that are linked with postherpetic neuralgia.

Additionally, garlic is an effective anti-inflammatory agent. There is a component in garlic called allicin, and research has shown that it can help decrease inflammation in the body. In addition to this, garlic is an excellent source of antioxidants, which are substances that help prevent harm to cells.

As a consequence of this, including garlic in your diet has the potential to assist in the alleviation of the discomfort and inflammation that are linked with postherpetic neuralgia.

Green Vegetables

The consumption of green vegetables is associated with improved nerve health because of their high nutritional content. The vitamins A, C, and E, together with the minerals potassium and magnesium, are included in this category.

Additionally, green veggies are an excellent way to obtain your fiber intake for the day. The digestive tract relies on fiber, which also has the added benefit of lowering inflammatory levels. You can help to enhance your general health and minimize your chance of getting postherpetic neuralgia by including green vegetables in your diet. This can be done in a way that is beneficial to both of these goals.

Fruits

The vitamin, mineral, and antioxidant content of fruits make them a valuable food source. These nutrients are necessary for maintaining healthy nerves and can aid in the reduction of inflammation that is brought on by postherpetic neuralgia.

Vitamin C, for instance, is required for the production of collagen, which in turn contributes to the good functioning of neurons. In addition, vitamin C is a potent antioxidant that helps to shield nerve cells from being damaged when they are exposed to free radicals.

In addition, the chemicals that are found in some fruits have been shown to have an anti-inflammatory impact. For instance, berries are a good source of anthocyanins, which have been found to lower the inflammatory response. Berries also include other beneficial antioxidants. Therefore, eating fruits daily may be beneficial for improving nerve health and reducing the symptoms of postherpetic neuralgia.

Whole Grains

Whole grains are particularly rich in fiber, as well as some vitamins and minerals. Both the health of the digestive tract and the inflammation brought on by postherpetic neuralgia may be improved by increasing fiber consumption.

Magnesium is essential for the metabolism of energy, the contraction of muscles, and the function of the nerves. Whole grains are an excellent source of magnesium. Additionally, magnesium has a role in the control of sugar levels in the blood. In addition, cancer and other chronic diseases may be avoided by eating whole grains since these grains contain phytochemicals, which can help prevent them.

You may help to enhance your general health and minimize your chance of getting postherpetic neuralgia by including these healthy items in your diet, which can also help improve your overall health.

Foods to Avoid

There is currently no known treatment for postherpetic neuralgia; however, there are several things that may be done to assist manage the symptoms of this condition. Avoiding items that might make the discomfort worse should be one of the most crucial things to keep in mind.

Foods high in carbohydrates

Inflammation is a potential side effect of consuming any diet that is rich in carbohydrate content. This is because the consumption of these meals causes an increase in the amount of sugar that is found in the blood. This, in turn, can cause nerve damage and make disorders like postherpetic neuralgia worse.

If you are experiencing symptoms of this disease, you must steer clear of the items listed above. Instead, you should make it a priority to consume foods that are low in carbohydrates and won't set off an inflammatory reaction in the body. You will find that doing so helps to reduce the severity of your symptoms and improves the overall quality of your life.

Foods high in saturated fats

Recent research has shown that there is a connection between inflammation and the kinds of nutrients that we take in via our diets. In particular, it would appear that saturated fats affect the development of inflammation. In addition to foods originating from animals, such as dairy and meat products, these fats can also be found in some oils derived from plants, such as cocoa butter, palm kernel oil, and coconut oil. These fats are present in dairy and meat products.

Other plant-based oils, such as olive oil, on the other hand, do not have any saturated fats in their composition. Even though further study has to be conducted in this field, it appears that eating meals that are heavy in saturated fats may make inflammation worse. People who are suffering from postherpetic neuralgia should steer clear of items that are classified into the aforementioned categories, which is why this piece of knowledge is so important to them.

Because of the connection between inflammation and nutrition, we can take actions to protect ourselves from experiencing future pain and suffering if we are aware of this connection.

Foods high in sugar

When taken in large quantities, sugar, which is a carbohydrate, is associated with the development of several undesirable health consequences. Inflammation is one of these undesirable side effects. When there is a sudden increase in the amount of sugar in the blood, this might lead to inflammation.

Sugary meals like sweets, cakes, and cookies can cause a sudden rise in blood sugar levels, which is undesirable for those who suffer from postherpetic neuralgia since these foods can induce a sharp rise in blood sugar levels.

As a result, persons who have this illness should steer clear of eating certain kinds of foods. They can aid in the prevention of inflammation and the sometimes debilitating pain that comes along with it by acting in this manner.

Processed foods

Inflammation and vitamin deficiency are only two of the health issues that have been associated with eating a diet that is high in processed foods. Sugar, salt, and bad fats are all widely present in processed meals, and these elements can increase inflammation.

In addition, processed foods frequently contain little nutrients, which means that consuming them regularly may result in vitamin shortages. If you are afflicted with postherpetic neuralgia, you must stay away from processed foods as much as you possibly can. You can help to minimize inflammation and enhance your general health if you follow a diet that is high in healthful whole foods.

Alcohol

Consumption of alcohol can have an effect that is directly related to postherpetic neuralgia. The inflammation that is connected with the ailment can be made worse by drinking significant amounts of alcohol, which can make the situation worse. This is because drinking alcohol may create an increase in the amount of sugar that is found in the blood, which in turn can cause an increase in the amount of inflammation that is present in the body.

Drinking alcohol can also lead to dehydration, which can be an additional factor that contributes to the inflammation that is brought on by postherpetic neuralgia. Because of this, those who are afflicted with postherpetic neuralgia are strongly encouraged to abstain from consuming alcoholic beverages.

Caffeine

Caffeine is widely acknowledged to have stimulant properties. To a lesser extent, however, people are aware that the same component that provides coffee with its energizing characteristics might also play a role in the development of inflammation. The effects of caffeine, in addition to the fact that it raises blood sugar levels, can ultimately increase inflammation.

Caffeine can induce an increase in blood sugar levels. In addition, caffeine can cause dehydration, which just makes the problem worse. Because of these factors, those who are afflicted with postherpetic neuralgia are strongly encouraged to refrain from drinking coffee.

If you suffer from postherpetic neuralgia, one of the most essential things you can do for yourself is to focus on eating a balanced diet. This requires a diet that is abundant in fruits, vegetables, whole cereals, and lean proteins.

You should also stay away from meals that have been processed, and foods that are high in sugar, alcohol, and caffeine. You may assist in lowering your chance of getting postherpetic neuralgia by adhering to this dietary advice, which can help you feel better faster.

If you are having difficulty controlling your pain, you might want to discuss possible pharmaceutical options with your primary care physician. Several different drugs may help provide pain relief for those suffering from postherpetic neuralgia.

Sample Recipes

Baked Flounder

Ingredients:

- 1 lb. flounder, fileted
- 1/4 tsp. salt
- 1 cup halved red grapes
- 1 tbsp. extra-virgin olive oil
- 2 tbsp. parsley, chopped finely
- 1 cup almonds, chopped and toasted
- freshly ground black pepper, to taste

Instructions:

1. Preheat the oven to 375°F.
2. Place fish on a sheet tray. Season with olive oil, salt, and pepper.
3. Combine the almonds, grapes, parsley, 1-1/2 tsp. of olive oil, 1/8 tsp of salt, and black pepper in a bowl.
4. Bake the fish for about 3 minutes.
5. Flip the fish and return to the oven.
6. Bake for another 3 minutes, or until the fish is starting to flake, while the center is still translucent. Don't overcook.
7. Serve immediately, topped with the grape mixture.

Asian-Themed Macrobiotic Bowl

Ingredients:

- 2 cups cooked quinoa
- 4 carrots
- 1 package of smoked tofu
- 1 tbsp. nutritional yeast
- 2 tbsp. coconut aminos
- 4 tbsp. sunflower sprouts
- 2 tbsp. fermented vegetables
- 1 cup of shiitake mushrooms
- 1 avocado
- 2 tbsp. hemp seeds
- 2-3 cooked beets
- coconut oil cooking spray

Dressing:

- 2 tbsp. miso paste
- 1 tbsp. tahini
- 1 tbsp. olive oil
- 3 tbsp. water

Instructions:

1. Roast the carrots in the oven at 400°F for 30-40 minutes.
2. Wash the vegetables, trim them, and spray them with coconut oil.

3. Add them to the oven. When they are cooked, set aside till you are ready to assemble the Buddha bowl.
4. Make the dressing by combining all of the ingredients in a medium-sized bowl. If the dressing appears lumpy, add more water.
5. To build the bowl, put the quinoa on the bottom and then arrange the vegetables on top.
6. Sprinkle the bowls with hemp seeds and drizzle the dressing over top.
7. Serve and enjoy.

Chicken Salad

Ingredients:

- 1 small can of premium chunk chicken breast packed in water
- 1 stalk celery, large, finely chopped
- 1/4 cup reduced-fat mayonnaise
- 4 romaine leaves or red leaf lettuce, washed and trimmed
- 1 cucumber, small and sliced thinly

Instructions:

1. Drain canned chicken and transfer to a bowl.
2. Put in celery and mayonnaise.
3. Mix lightly. Don't crush the chicken.
4. In a separate shallow bowl, place the lettuce neatly.
5. Add the chicken salad in the middle of the bowl.
6. Add cucumber slices to the plate.
7. Refrigerate before serving, cover with plastic wrap.

Baked Salmon

Ingredients:

- 2 salmon filets
- 6 cups of fresh spinach
- 2 tsp. coconut oil
- 1/4 tsp. turmeric
- salt
- pepper

Instructions:

1. Preheat the oven to 400°F.
2. Line a baking dish with parchment paper.
3. Marinate salmon filets coconut oil, turmeric, salt, and pepper.
4. Let it sit for a few minutes. This may also be done the night before to help the juices and flavor get into the salmon.
5. Once the oven is ready, bake the salmon for 15 minutes.
6. Add spinach and cook until ready. Season with salt and pepper to taste.
7. Take salmon out of the oven and put spinach beside it.
8. Serve and enjoy.

Asian Zucchini Salad

Ingredients:

- 1 medium zucchini, sliced thinly into spirals
- 1/3 cup rice vinegar
- 3/4 cup avocado oil
- 1 cup sunflower seeds, shells removed
- 1 lb. cabbage, shredded
- 1 tsp. stevia drops
- 1 cup almonds, sliced

Instructions:

1. Cut the zucchini spirals into smaller parts. Set aside.
2. Put almonds, sunflower seeds, and cabbage in a large bowl. Combine the ingredients well.
3. Add zucchini to the mixture.
4. In a small bowl, mix vinegar, stevia, and oil using a whisk or fork.
5. Pour the vinegar mixture all over the zucchini mixture. Toss well. Make sure everything is covered with the dressing.
6. Refrigerate for 2 hours before serving.

Low FODMAP Burger

Ingredients:

- 1-1/4 lbs. ground pork
- 1/2 tsp. salt
- 1/2 tsp. white pepper
- 1/2 tsp. ground nutmeg
- 1/2 tsp. caraway seeds
- 1/2 tsp. ground ginger

Instructions:

1. Preheat the grill then prepare the patty.
2. Using a small mixing bowl, stir together the salt, pepper, nutmeg, and ginger until fully combined.
3. Place the ground in a large mixing bowl and add the spice mixture.
4. Mix thoroughly until spices are evenly distributed to the pork.
5. Make round, flat burger patties using the palm of your hands.
6. Grill the patties and serve with gluten-free buns and mustard sauce.

Stir-Fried Cabbage and Apples

Ingredients:

- 1 shallot, thinly sliced
- 1/2 apple, cut into cubes
- 1/4 savoy cabbage, sliced thinly into strips
- 3–4 radishes, sliced thinly
- 1/2–1 tsp. coconut oil
- salt, to taste

Instructions:

1. Pour some coconut oil into a wok.
2. Add shallot and cook until translucent.
3. Add the cabbage, radish, and apples to the wok.
4. Stir-fry for about 5 minutes. Don't overcook.
5. Add salt to taste.
6. Serve while warm.

Asparagus and Greens Salad with Tahini and Poppy Seed Dressing

Ingredients:

- 10 to 12 asparagus stalks, washed well and sliced into ribbons
- 5 radishes, washed well and sliced thinly
- 2 to 3 rainbow carrots, peeled and sliced thinly
- 1 handful wild spinach
- 1 small handful of microgreens, washed well
- 1 small handful of sunflower greens, washed well
- optional: a few pieces of chive blossoms

For the dressing:

- 2 tbsp. tahini
- 1 tbsp. poppy seeds
- 1 tbsp. extra-virgin olive oil
- salt
- pepper

Instructions:

1. For the dressing, whisk ingredients together in a small bowl.
2. In a separate bowl, toss salad ingredients in the mixture.
3. Drizzle dressing on salad upon serving.

Roasted Chicken Thighs

Ingredients:

- 1 tbsp. avocado oil
- 1 pinch Himalayan pink salt
- 4 chicken thighs with skin
- 1 tsp. Primal Palate super gyro seasoning

Instructions:

1. Pour avocado oil over a medium-sized oven-safe pot.
2. Sauté over medium heat for 2 to 3 minutes or until the skins begin to brown.
3. Place the chicken in a large skillet over medium-high heat. Sear for about 2 to 3 minutes for each side, starting with the skin side.
4. Season generously with salt and Primal Palate Super Gyro seasoning.
5. Place the chicken in an oven preheated to 350°F.
6. Bake for one hour while covered.
7. Serve and enjoy.

Arugula and Mushroom Salad

Ingredients:

- 5 oz. arugula washed
- 1 lb. fresh mushrooms
- 1/4 tsp. shoyu
- 1 tbsp. olive oil
- 1 tbsp. mirin

For tofu cheese:

- 1/8 cup umeboshi vinegar
- 1/2 firm tofu

Instructions:

1. In a bowl, add the rinsed tofu. Crumble and pour in vinegar.
2. In a separate bowl add shoyu, salt, olive oil, and mirin. 3. Mix to combine.
3. Add in the arugula and toss to combine with the dressing.
4. Serve and enjoy.

Fresh Asparagus Salad

Ingredients:

- 1/3 cup of hazelnuts
- 4 cups arugula
- 1 tsp. ground pepper
- 2 tbsp. sea salt
- virgin olive oil
- 2 lbs. asparagus

Instructions:

1. Preheat the oven to 400°F.
2. Place hazelnuts on a baking tray with parchment paper. Place in the oven for 7 minutes.
3. Transfer hazelnuts to a plate. Optionally, to remove the skins, wrap the nuts in a towel and rub them vigorously.
4. Chop hazelnuts coarsely.
5. Remove the hard ends of the asparagus.
6. Place the stalks on the baking sheet you've used for the hazelnuts. Sprinkle 1 tbsp. olive oil and 1/2 tsp. of salt.
7. Bake for 8 minutes.
8. In a mixing bowl, combine pepper, salt, and olive oil. Mix well.

9. Place arugula in a medium bowl. Drizzle ½ of the dressing over the veggies. Toss until everything is well coated.
10. Place arugula onto a platter.
11. Arrange asparagus on top. Sprinkle peeled hazelnuts on top.

Tuna Salad

Ingredients:

- 1/2 cup pecans
- 1 cup chicken breast, steamed and cubed
- 1 cup tuna in oil
- salt, to taste
- pepper, to taste

Instructions:

1. Mix all ingredients in a large bowl.
2. Add a dash of salt and pepper to taste.
3. Chill for at least an hour before serving.

Conclusion

Postherpetic neuralgia, often known as PHN, is a disease that has the potential to develop in a patient after they have had chickenpox. It is possible for the chickenpox virus, which is responsible for the itchy, blistering rash that is associated with the childhood condition, to remain latent in a person's body for several years.

When the virus reactivates later in life as shingles, it has the potential to cause damage to the nerves, which can then lead to PHN. Intensely searing pain, heightened sensitivity to touch, and strong itching are some of the symptoms of PHN, which can be quite debilitating.

Postherpetic neuralgia is a disorder that causes excruciating pain and can be challenging to treat. On the other hand, there are certain things that you may do to assist in alleviating the symptoms of the condition. Eat a balanced diet and stay away from items that might make the pain even worse; this is one of the most important things to keep in mind.

You can make some strides in improving the quality of your life by putting these suggestions into practice. If the pain is severe, you should talk to a medical professional to see whether or not any additional therapies might be beneficial. On the other hand, you can significantly reduce the amount of discomfort you feel just by attending to your own needs.

References and Helpful Links

6 lifestyle tips for postherpetic neuralgia. (n.d.). Retrieved October 14, 2022, from https://patient.practicalpainmanagement.com/conditions/postherpetic-neuralgia/6-lifestyle-tips-postherpetic-neuralgia.

10 natural treatments and home remedies for shingles. (2018, June 14). https://www.medicalnewstoday.com/articles/322131.

ePainAssist, T. (2019, October 21). What to eat & avoid when you have postherpetic neuralgia? Epainassist. https://www.epainassist.com/diet-and-nutrition/what-to-eat-and-avoid-when-you-have-postherpetic-neuralgia.

Nutritional factors in herpes zoster, postherpetic neuralgia, and ... (n.d.). Retrieved October 14, 2022, from https://www.researchgate.net/publication/232609281_Nutritional_Factors_in_Herpes_Zoster_Postherpetic_Neuralgia_and_Zoster_Vaccination.

Post-herpetic neuralgia. (2018, October 3). Nhs.Uk. https://www.nhs.uk/conditions/post-herpetic-neuralgia/.

Postherpetic neuralgia: Symptoms, causes, treatment & prevention. (n.d.). Cleveland Clinic. Retrieved October 14, 2022, from https://my.clevelandclinic.org/health/diseases/12093-postherpetic-neuralgia.

What not to eat when you have shingles. (n.d.). EMedicineHealth. Retrieved October 14, 2022, from https://www.emedicinehealth.com/ask_what_not_to_eat_when_you_have_shingles/article_em.htm.

www.ingramcontent.com/pod-product-compliance
Lightning Source LLC
LaVergne TN
LVHW051924060526
838201LV00062B/4675